FATTY LIVER

COOKBOOK

RECIPES

For Newly Diagnosed

Jeffrey D. Mike

Contents

INTRODUCTION

Welcome to the ultimate guide to nourishing your liver and reclaiming your health! If you've recently been diagnosed with fatty liver disease, fret not, because I have crafted a deliciously rejuvenating cookbook tailored just for you.

Say goodbye to bland and boring meals, as we embark on a lip-smacking journey filled with flavors that will ignite your taste buds and ignite your liver's vitality.

In this fatty liver cookbook, I've handpicked a delightful assortment of recipes, meticulously designed to be low in fat yet bursting with essential nutrients.

My culinary masterpieces will not only tantalize your palate but also pave the way towards a healthier, happier you.

By adopting these liver-friendly recipes, you'll experience a myriad of benefits. First and foremost, these dishes are specifically crafted to reduce fat accumulation in your liver, promoting its healing and rejuvenation.

My carefully chosen ingredients, rich in antioxidants, vitamins, and minerals, will work together to combat oxidative stress, effectively protecting your liver from further damage.

Moreover, this cookbook is your gateway to improved overall health.

These nutrient-dense recipes will provide your body with the necessary fuel to enhance energy levels, support weight management, and boost your immune system – all vital factors for your liver's well-being.

But it doesn't stop there! The benefits of my fatty liver cookbook extend far beyond the kitchen. As you embrace the power of food as medicine, you'll discover a newfound sense of empowerment and control over your health journey.

With each delicious meal, you'll be nourishing not only your body but also your mind, uplifting your spirits as you witness positive changes unfolding.

Whether you're a seasoned chef or a cooking novice, these recipes are thoughtfully curated to be easy-to-follow and time-friendly, ensuring that your path to a healthier liver is as effortless as it is delicious.

Embrace the power of food as medicine, and let's embark on this flavorful adventure together.

So, grab your apron, sharpen those knives, and let's cook our way to a revitalized liver and a brighter tomorrow! Your health is your greatest wealth, and this cookbook is your key to unlock a world of well-being and vitality.

Let's savor every mouthwatering moment as we take charge of our liver health and embrace a life of wellness.

RECIPES

GRILLED SALMON WITH LEMON AND DILL

Ingredients

- Fresh salmon fillets
- Fresh dill
- Lemon juice
- Olive oil
- Salt and pepper

Preparation

- Preheat the grill to medium-high heat.
- Season the salmon fillets with salt and pepper.
- Mix fresh dill, lemon juice, and olive oil to create a marinade.

- Coat the salmon fillets with the marinade and let them sit for about 15-30 minutes.
- Grill the salmon for about 4-5 minutes per side or until cooked through.

BAKED COD WITH HERBS

Ingredients

- Fresh cod fillets
- Fresh herbs (such as thyme, rosemary, and parsley)
- Lemon juice
- Olive oil
- Salt and pepper

Preparation

- Preheat the oven to 400°F (200°C).
- Season the cod fillets with salt and pepper.

- Mix fresh herbs, lemon juice, and olive oil to create a marinade.

- Coat the cod fillets with the marinade and let them sit for about 15-30 minutes.

- Place the cod fillets on a baking sheet lined with parchment paper and bake for about 15-20 minutes or until the fish is flaky.

LEMON GARLIC SHRIMP SKEWERS

Ingredients

- Fresh shrimp, peeled and deveined
- Lemon juice
- Minced garlic
- Olive oil
- Salt and pepper

Preparation

- Preheat the grill or grill pan to medium-high heat.

- Thread the shrimp onto skewers.

- Mix lemon juice, minced garlic, olive oil, salt, and pepper to create a marinade.

- Coat the shrimp skewers with the marinade and let them sit for about 10-15 minutes.

- Grill the shrimp skewers for about 2-3 minutes per side or until they are pink and cooked through.

TURKEY AND VEGETABLE STIR-FRY

Ingredients

- Lean ground turkey
- Sliced bell peppers (assorted colors)
- Sliced carrots
- Snap peas

- Soy sauce (low-sodium)

- Minced ginger

- Minced garlic

- Olive oil

Preparation

- In a large pan or wok, heat olive oil over medium-high heat.

- Add minced ginger and garlic and stir-fry for about 1 minute until fragrant.

- Add the ground turkey and cook until browned.

- Add the sliced vegetables and stir-fry until they are tender-crisp.

- Pour in low-sodium soy sauce and continue to stir-fry for another minute.

- Serve the stir-fry over brown rice or cauliflower rice.

LENTIL AND VEGETABLE SOUP

Ingredients

- Red lentils
- Chopped onions
- Sliced carrots
- Chopped celery
- Low-sodium vegetable broth
- Turmeric
- Ground cumin
- Fresh parsley

Preparation

- In a large pot, sauté the chopped onions, carrots, and celery until they are softened.
- Add red lentils, vegetable broth, turmeric, and ground cumin to the pot.

- Bring the mixture to a boil, then reduce the heat and simmer until the lentils are cooked and the vegetables are tender.
- Stir in fresh parsley before serving.

QUINOA STUFFED BELL PEPPERS

Ingredients

- Bell peppers (assorted colors)
- Cooked quinoa
- Chopped onions
- Chopped tomatoes
- Cooked black beans
- Ground cumin
- Paprika
- Salt and pepper

Preparation

- Preheat the oven to 375°F (190°C).

- Cut the tops off the bell peppers and remove the seeds and membranes.

- In a bowl, mix cooked quinoa, chopped onions, chopped tomatoes, and cooked black beans.

- Season the mixture with ground cumin, paprika, salt, and pepper.

- Stuff the bell peppers with the quinoa mixture and place them in a baking dish.

- Bake for about 20-25 minutes or until the peppers are tender.

CHICKPEA AND SPINACH CURRY

Ingredients

- Cooked chickpeas
- Fresh spinach leaves
- Diced tomatoes
- Chopped onions
- Minced garlic
- Minced ginger
- Curry powder
- Cumin powder
- Turmeric powder
- Coconut milk (light or low-fat)
- Olive oil
- Salt and pepper

Preparation

- In a large pan, sauté the chopped onions, minced garlic, and minced ginger until fragrant.

- Add diced tomatoes and cook until they soften.

- Stir in curry powder, cumin powder, and turmeric powder and cook for another minute.

- Add cooked chickpeas and fresh spinach leaves to the pan.

- Pour in light coconut milk and let the mixture simmer until the spinach wilts and the flavors meld.

- Season with salt and pepper to taste.

GRILLED CHICKEN WITH HERBS

Ingredients

- Skinless chicken breasts
- Fresh herbs (such as thyme, rosemary, and oregano)
- Lemon juice
- Olive oil
- Salt and pepper

Preparation

- Preheat the grill to medium-high heat.
- Season the chicken breasts with salt and pepper.
- Mix fresh herbs, lemon juice, and olive oil to create a marinade.
- Coat the chicken breasts with the marinade and let them sit for about 15-30 minutes.

- Grill the chicken for about 4-5 minutes per side or until cooked through.

TOFU AND BROCCOLI STIR-FRY

Ingredients

- Firm tofu, cubed
- Broccoli florets
- Sliced bell peppers (assorted colors)
- Soy sauce (low-sodium)
- Minced ginger
- Minced garlic
- Sesame oil
- Olive oil

Preparation

- In a large pan or wok, heat olive oil over medium-high heat.

- Add minced ginger and garlic and stir-fry for about 1 minute until fragrant.

- Add cubed tofu and stir-fry until lightly browned.

- Add broccoli florets and sliced bell peppers and continue to stir-fry until they are tender-crisp.

- Pour in low-sodium soy sauce and a dash of sesame oil and stir-fry for another minute.

- Serve the tofu and broccoli stir-fry over brown rice or quinoa.

BAKED SWEET POTATOES WITH OLIVE OIL AND HERBS

Ingredients

- Sweet potatoes
- Olive oil
- Dried herbs (such as rosemary, thyme, and paprika)
- Salt and pepper

Preparation

- Preheat the oven to 400°F (200°C).
- Scrub the sweet potatoes and pierce them with a fork several times.
- Rub olive oil over the sweet potatoes and sprinkle with dried herbs, salt, and pepper.
- Place the sweet potatoes on a baking sheet lined with parchment paper.

- Bake for about 45-60 minutes or until the sweet potatoes are tender when pierced with a fork.

GREEK YOGURT WITH BERRIES AND NUTS

Ingredients

- Greek yogurt (low-fat or fat-free)
- Mixed berries (blueberries, raspberries, strawberries)
- Chopped nuts (such as almonds or walnuts)

Preparation

- In a bowl, place a generous scoop of Greek yogurt.
- Top the yogurt with mixed berries and chopped nuts.

MIXED BERRY SMOOTHIE

Ingredients

- Mixed berries (blueberries, raspberries, strawberries)
- Low-fat yogurt
- Almond milk
- Honey (optional)

Preparation

- In a blender, combine mixed berries, low-fat yogurt, and almond milk.
- Blend until smooth and add honey for sweetness if desired.

SPINACH AND MUSHROOM FRITTATA

Ingredients

- Fresh spinach leaves
- Sliced mushrooms
- Chopped onions
- Eggs
- Milk
- Grated Parmesan cheese (optional)
- Olive oil
- Salt and pepper

Preparation

- In an oven-safe skillet, sauté chopped onions and sliced mushrooms in olive oil until tender.

- Add fresh spinach leaves to the skillet and cook until wilted.

- In a bowl, whisk eggs, milk, salt, and pepper. Pour the mixture over the vegetables.

- Sprinkle grated Parmesan cheese on top (optional).

- Bake in a preheated oven at 375°F (190°C) for about 15-20 minutes or until the frittata is set.

ROASTED BRUSSELS SPROUTS WITH BALSAMIC GLAZE

Ingredients

- Brussels sprouts

- Olive oil

- Balsamic glaze or vinegar

- Salt and pepper

Preparation

- Preheat the oven to 400°F (200°C).

- Trim and halve Brussels sprouts, if large.

- Toss Brussels sprouts with olive oil, salt, and pepper.

- Roast in the oven for about 20-25 minutes until they are crispy and caramelized.

- Drizzle balsamic glaze or vinegar over the roasted Brussels sprouts before serving.

CAULIFLOWER RICE PILAF WITH ALMONDS

Ingredients

- Cauliflower rice (pre-packaged or homemade)

- Sliced almonds

- Chopped onions

- Chopped carrots

- Olive oil

- Fresh parsley

- Salt and pepper

Preparation

- In a pan, sauté chopped onions and chopped carrots in olive oil until softened.

- Add cauliflower rice to the pan and cook until tender.

- Mix in sliced almonds, fresh parsley, salt, and pepper before serving.

TOMATO AND CUCUMBER SALAD WITH FETA

Ingredients

- Chopped tomatoes
- Sliced cucumbers
- Crumbled feta cheese (in moderation)
- Chopped red onions
- Fresh parsley
- Olive oil
- Lemon juice
- Salt and pepper

Preparation

- In a bowl, combine chopped tomatoes, sliced cucumbers, crumbled feta cheese, and chopped red onions.

- Drizzle olive oil and lemon juice over the salad.

- Sprinkle fresh parsley, salt, and pepper and toss to combine.

KALE AND CHICKPEA SALAD

Ingredients

- Chopped kale leaves

- Cooked chickpeas

- Chopped bell peppers (assorted colors)

- Chopped red onions

- Sunflower seeds (optional)

- Olive oil

- Lemon juice

- Salt and pepper

Preparation

- In a large bowl, combine chopped kale leaves, cooked chickpeas, chopped bell peppers, and chopped red onions.

- If desired, add sunflower seeds for extra crunch.

- Dress the salad with olive oil, lemon juice, salt, and pepper. Toss to combine.

AVOCADO AND TOMATO SALAD

Ingredients

- Diced avocados

- Chopped tomatoes

- Chopped red onions

- Fresh cilantro or parsley

- Lime juice

- Olive oil

- Salt and pepper

Preparation

- In a bowl, gently mix diced avocados, chopped tomatoes, and chopped red onions.

- Add fresh cilantro or parsley for added flavor.

- Dress the salad with lime juice, olive oil, salt, and pepper. Toss gently to avoid mashing the avocados.

BROCCOLI AND WALNUT SALAD

Ingredients

- Fresh broccoli florets

- Chopped walnuts

- Dried cranberries (in moderation)

- Red wine vinegar

- Olive oil

- Dijon mustard

- Honey (optional)

- Salt and pepper

Preparation

- Steam or blanch fresh broccoli florets until tender-crisp.

- In a bowl, combine steamed broccoli, chopped walnuts, and dried cranberries (if using).

- In a separate bowl, whisk red wine vinegar, olive oil, Dijon mustard, honey (if using), salt, and pepper to make the dressing.

- Pour the dressing over the salad and toss to coat.

CARROT AND CILANTRO SALAD

Ingredients

- Grated carrots
- Fresh cilantro
- Lemon juice
- Olive oil
- Ground cumin
- Salt and pepper

Preparation

- In a bowl, combine grated carrots and chopped fresh cilantro.
- Dress the salad with lemon juice, olive oil, ground cumin, salt, and pepper. Toss to combine.

BROWN RICE AND BLACK BEAN BURRITO BOWL

Ingredients

- Cooked brown rice
- Cooked black beans
- Sliced bell peppers (assorted colors)
- Sliced avocado
- Chopped red onions
- Fresh cilantro
- Lime juice
- Olive oil
- Salt and pepper

Preparation

- In a bowl, layer cooked brown rice, cooked black beans, and sliced bell peppers.

- Top the bowl with sliced avocado and chopped red onions.

- Dress the burrito bowl with fresh cilantro, lime juice, olive oil, salt, and pepper.

ZUCCHINI NOODLES WITH TURKEY BOLOGNESE SAUCE

Ingredients

- Zucchini noodles (zoodles)

- Lean ground turkey

- Chopped onions

- Chopped carrots

- Crushed tomatoes

- Minced garlic

- Olive oil

- Fresh basil

- Salt and pepper

Preparation

- In a large pan, heat olive oil over medium heat and sauté chopped onions, chopped carrots, and minced garlic until softened.
- Add lean ground turkey and cook until browned.
- Pour crushed tomatoes into the pan and simmer until the sauce thickens.
- Season the sauce with fresh basil, salt, and pepper.
- Serve the Bolognese sauce over zucchini noodles.

MISO SOUP WITH TOFU AND WAKAME

Ingredients

- Miso paste

- Silken tofu, cubed

- Wakame seaweed

- Sliced green onions

- Dashi broth (or vegetable broth)

- Water

- Soy sauce (low-sodium) – optional

Preparation

- In a pot, combine water and dashi broth and bring to a simmer.

- Add cubed silken tofu and wakame seaweed to the pot.

- In a small bowl, mix miso paste with a little hot water to form a paste, then add it to the pot.

- Simmer the soup gently, making sure not to boil the miso, as it can lose its flavor.

- If desired, add a splash of low-sodium soy sauce for additional seasoning.

- Garnish the soup with sliced green onions before serving.

ROASTED BEET AND ARUGULA SALAD

Ingredients

- Roasted beets, sliced

- Fresh arugula leaves

- Crumbled goat cheese (in moderation)

- Chopped walnuts

- Balsamic glaze or vinegar

- Olive oil

- Salt and pepper

Preparation

- Preheat the oven to 400°F (200°C).

- Wrap whole beets in aluminum foil and roast them for about 40-60 minutes until tender.

- Let the beets cool, then peel and slice them.

- In a bowl, combine fresh arugula leaves, sliced roasted beets, crumbled goat cheese, and chopped walnuts.

- Dress the salad with balsamic glaze or vinegar, olive oil, salt, and pepper. Toss to combine.

STEAMED ASPARAGUS WITH LEMON

Ingredients

- Fresh asparagus spears

- Lemon wedges

- Olive oil

- Salt and pepper

Preparation

- Trim the tough ends of the asparagus spears.
- Steam the asparagus in a steamer basket or by placing them in a pan with a small amount of water and covering with a lid.
- Steam for about 4-5 minutes until the asparagus is tender-crisp.
- Drizzle with olive oil and season with salt and pepper.
- Serve with lemon wedges on the side for squeezing over the asparagus.

BAKED APPLES WITH CINNAMON

Ingredients

- Apples (such as Honeycrisp or Gala)
- Ground cinnamon
- Honey (optional)

Preparation

- Preheat the oven to 375°F (190°C).
- Core the apples and cut a small slit around the middle to prevent bursting.
- Sprinkle ground cinnamon over the apples, and if desired, drizzle a little honey inside the core.
- Place the apples in a baking dish and bake for about 20-25 minutes or until they are tender.

GINGER GARLIC BAKED CHICKEN THIGHS

Ingredients

- Bone-in, skin-on chicken thighs
- Minced ginger
- Minced garlic
- Soy sauce (low-sodium)
- Honey (optional)
- Olive oil
- Salt and pepper

Preparation

- In a bowl, mix minced ginger, minced garlic, low-sodium soy sauce, and olive oil to make a marinade.
- If desired, add honey for sweetness.

- Coat the chicken thighs with the marinade and let them marinate in the refrigerator for at least 30 minutes.

- Preheat the oven to 400°F (200°C).

- Place the marinated chicken thighs on a baking sheet lined with parchment paper.

- Bake for about 25-30 minutes or until the chicken is cooked through and the skin is crispy.

GARLIC ROASTED CAULIFLOWER

Ingredients

- Fresh cauliflower florets
- Minced garlic
- Olive oil
- Lemon juice
- Paprika
- Salt and pepper

Preparation

- Preheat the oven to 425°F (220°C).

- In a bowl, toss cauliflower florets with minced garlic, olive oil, and lemon juice.

- Sprinkle with paprika, salt, and pepper, and toss to coat evenly.

- Spread the cauliflower on a baking sheet lined with parchment paper.

- Roast for about 25-30 minutes or until the cauliflower is golden and tender.

BERRY CHIA PUDDING

Ingredients

- Chia seeds

- Almond milk

- Mixed berries (blueberries, raspberries, strawberries)

- Honey (optional)

Preparation

- In a bowl, mix chia seeds and almond milk. Stir well to prevent clumping.
- Let the mixture sit for about 5-10 minutes to thicken.
- If desired, add honey for sweetness.
- Layer chia pudding with mixed berries in a serving glass or jar.
- Refrigerate for at least 2 hours or overnight before serving.

VEGETABLE OMELETTE WITH FRESH HERBS

Ingredients

- Eggs
- Chopped bell peppers (assorted colors)
- Chopped onions
- Chopped tomatoes
- Fresh herbs (such as parsley, chives, or basil)
- Olive oil
- Salt and pepper

Preparation

- In a bowl, whisk eggs with a pinch of salt and pepper.

- In a non-stick pan, sauté chopped bell peppers and chopped onions in olive oil until softened.

- Pour the beaten eggs over the vegetables and cook until the omelette is set.

- Before folding the omelette, add chopped tomatoes and fresh herbs for added freshness and flavor.

- Fold the omelette in half and serve warm.

MEAL PLAN

DAY 1

Breakfast: Spinach and Mushroom Frittata

Lunch: Lentil and Vegetable Soup

Dinner: Grilled Salmon with Lemon and Dill, served with Steamed Asparagus with Lemon

DAY 2

Breakfast: Greek Yogurt with Berries and Nuts

Lunch: Chickpea and Spinach Curry

Dinner: Zucchini Noodles with Turkey Bolognese Sauce

DAY 3

Breakfast: Berry Chia Pudding

Lunch: Roasted Brussels Sprouts with Balsamic Glaze, served with Quinoa Stuffed Bell Peppers

Dinner: Baked Cod with Herbs, served with Cauliflower Rice Pilaf with Almonds

DAY 4

Breakfast: Vegetable Omelette with Fresh Herbs

Lunch: Mixed Berry Smoothie

Dinner: Tofu and Broccoli Stir-Fry, served with Brown Rice and Black Bean Burrito Bowl

DAY 5

Breakfast: Baked Apples with Cinnamon

Lunch: Avocado and Tomato Salad, served with Garlic Roasted Cauliflower

Dinner: Lemon Garlic Shrimp Skewers, served with Kale and Chickpea Salad

DAY 6

Breakfast: Quinoa Stuffed Bell Peppers

Lunch: Lentil and Vegetable Soup

Dinner: Grilled Chicken with Herbs, served with Roasted Beet and Arugula Salad

DAY 7

Breakfast: Greek Yogurt with Berries and Nuts

Lunch: Miso Soup with Tofu and Wakame, served with Tomato and Cucumber Salad with Feta

Dinner: Chickpea and Spinach Curry, served with Cauliflower Rice Pilaf with Almonds

DAY 8

Breakfast: Berry Chia Pudding

Lunch: Baked Sweet Potatoes with Olive Oil and Herbs, served with Broccoli and Walnut Salad

Dinner: Tofu and Broccoli Stir-Fry, served with Brown Rice and Black Bean Burrito Bowl

DAY 9

Breakfast: Vegetable Omelette with Fresh Herbs

Lunch: Grilled Salmon with Lemon and Dill, served with Steamed Asparagus with Lemon

Dinner: Lemon Garlic Shrimp Skewers, served with Kale and Chickpea Salad

DAY 10

Breakfast: Mixed Berry Smoothie

Lunch: Roasted Brussels Sprouts with Balsamic Glaze, served with Quinoa Stuffed Bell Peppers

Dinner: Baked Cod with Herbs, served with Roasted Beet and Arugula Salad

DAY 11

Breakfast: Baked Apples with Cinnamon

Lunch: Avocado and Tomato Salad, served with Garlic Roasted Cauliflower

Dinner: Grilled Chicken with Herbs, served with Tomato and Cucumber Salad with Feta

DAY 12

Breakfast: Quinoa Stuffed Bell Peppers

Lunch: Lentil and Vegetable Soup

Dinner: Zucchini Noodles with Turkey Bolognese Sauce

DAY 13

Breakfast: Greek Yogurt with Berries and Nuts

Lunch: Chickpea and Spinach Curry, served with Cauliflower Rice Pilaf with Almonds

Dinner: Tofu and Broccoli Stir-Fry, served with Brown Rice and Black Bean Burrito Bowl

DAY 14

Breakfast: Berry Chia Pudding

Lunch: Miso Soup with Tofu and Wakame, served with Broccoli and Walnut Salad

Dinner: Grilled Salmon with Lemon and Dill, served with Steamed Asparagus with Lemon

CONCLUSION

"Fatty Liver Cookbook for the Newly Diagnosed" is not just a collection of recipes; it's a guiding light, a companion, and a source of hope for your newfound journey to wellness.

As you embrace this culinary adventure, remember that you hold the power to nourish your body and take charge of your liver health.

From the vibrant flavors that dance on your taste buds to the knowledge that empowers your understanding, this cookbook is a testament to the resilience of the human spirit.

With each delicious dish you create, you are forging a path towards a healthier, happier tomorrow.

Together, we stand as a community of support, where experiences are shared, and triumphs are celebrated. So, let this cookbook be your ally, your inspiration, and your ticket to a brighter future.

Today marks a new beginning—a chapter filled with flavors, nourishment, and possibilities. Embrace the journey ahead with confidence and courage, knowing that you have the tools to savor life and embrace the richness of health.

So, turn up the heat, unleash your inner chef, and embark on this flavorful expedition hand in hand with "Fatty Liver Cookbook for the Newly Diagnosed."

Embrace the delicious delights that await you and discover the joy of nourishing your body from the inside out.

Welcome to a world of healing and culinary bliss—your wellness is now in your hands.

Let's savor the moments, cherish the flavors, and celebrate a life well-lived, one liver-loving recipe at a time.

Here's to a future filled with health, happiness, and a cookbook that will forever be your ally on this incredible journey!

9 798854 206266